Author and editor: Sarah Plater
Illustrator and designer: Sophie Carpenter

Typefaces: Avenir (© Adrian Frutiger), Engine (© Ferdie Balderas)
Printed in: Willersey, England by Vale Press

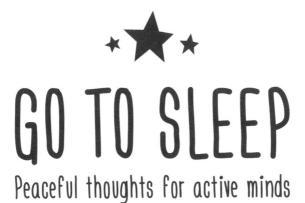

GO TO SLEEP

Peaceful thoughts for active minds

CONTENTS

INTRODUCTION

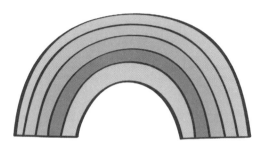

Irish legend has it that there is a pot of gold at the end of every rainbow. The myth endures because you can never reach the end. Every time you move closer, the rainbow shifts further into the distance. At times in everyone's life, falling asleep seems just as elusive.

In most things, increased effort brings improved results. Sleep is the exception. The more we try to sleep, the more impossible it becomes.

The transition from wakefulness to slumber is like a light switch we cannot reach. Trying to make ourselves fall asleep is as outside of our control as trying to change how our fingernails grow.

Imagine you are making bread. You mix the flour, yeast, oil and water together. Then you need to step back and let nature continue the process by making the dough rise.

It's the same with sleep. There are things you can do to prepare you for sleep. Beyond that, you need to trust in the natural process of falling asleep. That's why our recipe for preparing for a restful night has just three ingredients:

- Following the Good Sleep Habits

- Winding down and preparing for bed

- Calming your mind once in bed

All of these things are under your control. Focus on bringing them together, and then let your body take care of the final transition to sleep, without pressuring yourself.

Part I of this book will show you the Six Good Sleep Habits that will ensure your body feels tired. Implement these immediately. As you re-gain the ability to sleep effortlessly, you can experiment to see which habits have the biggest impact for you, and be more flexible with the rest of them.

Part II suggests some ways you can wind down as part of your evening routine. This helps to prepare your body and mind for rest by switching off from the worries and cares of your day.

Part III shows you a range of techniques to relax your mind. Each week, just before you get into bed, choose which one of these techniques to try. Our brains can be distracted by the novelty of doing something new, so try each technique for the whole week before making a decision as to whether or not it helped you. If you found it relaxing, mark that page so you can come back to it. Over time, you will learn which techniques work for you in different situations.

At first, you may find that your mind keeps drifting back to your worries. Simply notice that this has happened and gently bring your focus back to the technique you are trying. Repeat as necessary. With practice, your focus will improve.

Adopt the Good Sleep Habits, wind down before bed and learn the techniques to relax your mind. Don't worry about - or try to control - anything else. Soon you will find that going to sleep is the easiest, most pleasant and most natural thing in the world. And the rediscovery of effortless sleep is even more valuable than finding a pot of gold at the end of the rainbow.

Health conditions

If you have a health condition, the natural process of falling asleep may require medical assistance. Always seek professional advice.

HOW TO USE THIS BOOK

1. Follow the Six Good Sleep Habits, described in **Part I**.

2. Relax and unwind before going to bed. Suggestions for doing this can be found in **Part II**.

3. Follow a technique or use a visualisation to calm your mind while you're in bed. These can be found in **Part III**.

Try each technique and visualisation several times before making a judgement about its effectiveness. At first, the novelty of trying something new can cause your brain to become more alert, because our brains focus on anything unfamiliar as a defence mechanism. After a week or so of use, the technique will feel familiar and you are likely to find that you sleep much better than before you used it.

Mixed in throughout the book are calming quotes that will support you to move towards an improved, positive relationship with your sleep.

PART I

The Six Good Sleep Habits

Follow these six habits to ensure your body feels tired by bedtime. Start implementing them into your life immediately. Sleep is a very individual thing, so you may find that some of the habits are more essential to you than others. To begin with, keep to all of them, then gradually experiment with them over time to find out which ones you can be more flexible about.

1. Maintain a sleep routine

Train your body when to wake and when to sleep by keeping to a routine. If you go out one evening, get up at your usual time the next day to avoid confusing your body's sleep rhythm. Don't deviate from your routine by more than half an hour, even on Sunday mornings - it will be worth it!

If you wake feeling tired, don't think about it or tell everyone what a bad sleeper you are - both of these things make you feel worse, and contribute to unhelpful beliefs about your ability to sleep.

These unhelpful beliefs can be the reason why you struggle to sleep in the first place: you've trained your brain that sleep is something that is difficult to do. That makes you unable to relax and you lose trust in your ability to fall asleep.

Learn to regain that trust, keep a routine and use a relaxation technique to help distract your mind. Soon sleep won't be an issue for you anymore.

If you want to fall asleep earlier in the evening, get up 15 minutes earlier each day, until you are tired at the desired time. Do you struggle to get out of bed? Plan something you're excited about doing for those first 15 minutes, or put your alarm clock on the other side of the room to force you to leave the bed.

Stay in bed for the number of hours of sleep you need, but no more. How much sleep you need is an individual thing; from as little as four hours to as many as ten. As a starting point, aim for eight hours in bed. Decrease this time if you find yourself awake for long parts of it; increase the time if you are asleep for all of it and still feel tired. The amount needed decreases as we get older - accept this and don't try to sleep for longer than you need.

What about naps? Some people can nap during the day without affecting their night-time sleep, others can't. If in doubt, avoid naps.

2. Wind down before bedtime

Gradually decrease your activity levels in the 90-minute lead-up to your bedtime. Lower the lights and get ready for bed, just as you spend time preparing for other elements of your life.

Put your phone on airplane mode and leave it out of reach to avoid the temptation of reacting to that flashing notifications light. Use an old style alarm clock to wake you up instead. Turn off your television and put your tablet away (the type of light emitted from these devices can keep you wakeful).

Avoid caffeinated drinks after lunch, or smoking within four hours of sleeping. An occasional alcoholic drink is fine, but drinking a lot can reduce the quality of the sleep you get. Avoid eating heavy meals, chocolate or sugar within a few hours of your bedtime.

Turn to **Part II** for more ideas on how to wind down and prepare for bed.

3. Create a sleep-friendly environment

Use your bed (and your bedroom, if possible) only for sleeping. This helps your brain to associate that space with rest and relaxation. Use these tips to make the room as conducive to sleep as possible:

- Aim for a room temperature of around 15-20°C.

- Use thick curtains or blackout blinds to darken the space as much as possible.

- Remove light sources (e.g. LEDs from electronic devices) and if you need a clock in the room, use one you can't see when the lights are off or turn/hide the screen.

- Wear loose, comfortable pyjamas or sleep naked.

- Make sure you feel comfortable in bed. That might mean investing in a better mattress, or using a pillow underneath your legs (for back sleepers) or between your knees (for side sleepers).

- Use earplugs if your partner snores, if there's loud traffic nearby or noise from people or animals outside.

4. Look after yourself

A healthy diet ensures your body gets the nutrients it needs to create sleep-promoting hormones. Eat fresh, varied, unprocessed food including a range of vegetable, seeds and nuts. A secondary benefit is that eating better makes you feel better. You'll do more during the day as a result, and thus feel more tired and ready to sleep at night.

Get sunlight on your face during the morning to encourage your body to secrete the right hormones at the right time of day. This can be as simple as taking a walk around the block when you first wake up, getting off the bus a stop early, or stretching your legs before going into work. Spending time in nature has many secondary benefits on your mood and health, so head for a local park or a bit of countryside if you can.

Find some exercise you enjoy and do it regularly. Try to get 20-30 minutes of exercise every day, even if that's just a walk. Commit to doing this even if you feel tired right now - you will feel better for it afterwards!

5. Practice calming techniques

Practice mindfulness and meditation during the day. The more comfortable and confident you get with reacting calmly to your thoughts, feelings and emotions, the more successfully you will be able to do it at night. It takes practice, but learning to control how you respond to what's going on in your head will change your life beyond just improving your sleep quality.

Mindfulness just means being aware of what you are experiencing right now. It's about paying attention to your five senses and noticing the thoughts, feelings and emotions you are having. You can notice worries, identify them and let them pass, without feeling that you need to act on them or respond to them.

Meditation can take several forms. Guided meditations take you on a peaceful mental journey. Breathing meditation is about noticing and following your breathing pattern. Movement-based meditation includes mindful physical activity such as yoga.

6. Focus on living your life

At some points in your life, you have fallen asleep straight away, with no effort on your part. You didn't need to control everything in your life to achieve it. So stop putting your life on hold: it's counterproductive. Sleep is not a problem to be solved. Accept that everyone occasionally sleeps less than they'd like - and that's fine!

Sleep (or perceived lack of it) is not something to be feared, dreaded and controlled. Indeed, thinking negatively about sleep is often the root cause of the problem.

If you avoid going out with your friends in the evenings, insist on sleeping separately from your partner and spend all day plotting and planning how you will sleep tonight, you will amplify your sleep problems.

This is because you are training yourself to be anxious about sleep and how you can control it. You can't control it. You can only re-learn to trust your natural ability to fall asleep.

Follow all of these sleep habits when you can, but be willing to be flexible. Don't panic if you occasionally eat an unhealthy meal out with friends late in the evening.

Get on with living, use this book to help you relax at night, and sleep will soon follow. Trust the process, and trust your body to do its thing without letting your mind get in the way.

PART II

Wind down and prepare for bed

Insert a buffer between your busy day and your bedtime. The 90 minutes or so before you climb into bed are time for you to unwind and prepare your body for sleep.

You could opt for a warm bath, a good novel or follow one of the suggestions in this part of the book.

This section also provides ideas for making your sleep space as welcoming and relaxing as possible, so you start looking forward to going to bed each night.

O

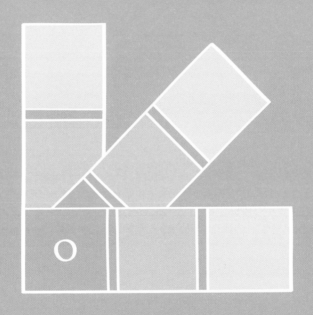

#1 Blue: the sleep hue

Rest your eyes on shades of blue, like those used in this book. It's known to be a mentally calming and soothing colour. One study showed that people with blue bedrooms slept longer than people in rooms with other colours.

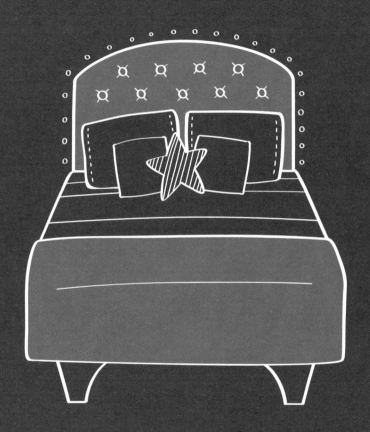

#2 Invest in your bed

Make it a place you love to retreat to. Spend time trying out all the mattresses in the store, and choose the one you don't want to get up from. Splurge on silky pillowcases and cosy duvets in natural fabrics - cool linen in summer, combed cotton in winter.

As businessman George Glasgow Jr said, "You should invest heavily in your bed and your shoes, because if you're not in one then you're in the other."

#3 A time to worry; a time to rest

Allow yourself time before bed (and outside of the bedroom) to think through your worries and decide what to take action on and what to make peace with.

If those worries trespass into your thoughts later when you are in bed, remind yourself 'this is my time for rest'.

"Don't try to solve serious matters
in the middle of the night."

PHILIP K. DICK
American writer (1928 – 1982)

#4 De-stress with a card game

Get a deck of cards and play some card games to take your mind off other things.

If you have a partner or flatmate, you could play Pairs or Rummy. For solo play, try Solitaire, Elevens or even try building a house of cards.

#5 Have a cuddle

The hormone oxytocin is produced when we have skin to skin contact with others. This hormone has been linked to helping us bond, relax and sleep, so make cuddling up with your loved ones part of your wind-down ritual.

Stay in the present and make it a mindful experience by focusing on every detail of how it feels to be close to someone you care about - what you feel, smell and see during those moments.

#6 Stretch and relax with yoga

Multiple studies have linked yoga with sleep benefits.
Follow the routine on the next few pages each night
before getting in bed. Hold each pose for five inhalations
and exhalations. Keep all stretches at a comfortable
intensity for your level of fitness.

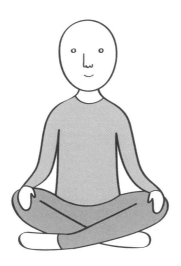

1. Breathing slow-down

Sit cross-legged, with your back straight and your hands resting lightly on your knees. If this isn't comfortable, place a folded towel under your bum. Turn your attention to your natural breathing, then start to lengthen your inhalations and exhalations. Breathe in and out through your nose and feel each breath fill your stomach.

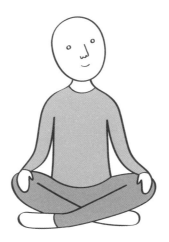

2. Neck rolls

Move your hands to your hips, and breathe in as you gently rotate your head in a loop: dip your chin as you look down and then to the left. Tilt your right ear to the ceiling, gradually tipping your head back and to the left. Breathe out as you continue the loop around the right side of your body. Do this twice, then repeat in the other direction. Keep your shoulders low and relaxed throughout.

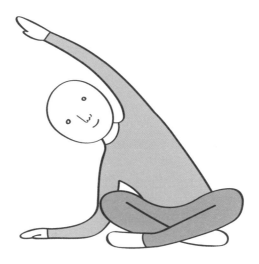

3. Side stretch

Place your left arm out on the floor, a little way away
from the left side of your body. Slowly stretch your right
arm out to the right, then bring it over your head and
towards the left side of your body, letting your head lean
to the left. Both of your sit bones should stay firmly on
the floor at all times. Repeat on the other side.

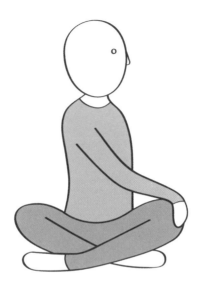

4. Seated twist

Put your right hand on the outside of your left thigh and move your left hand out behind you. Twist to look over your left shoulder, keeping your back straight. Stretch taller as you breathe in, and twist a little further as you breathe out. Repeat on the other side.

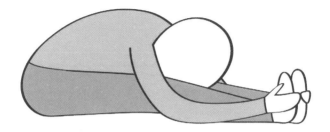

5. Forward bends

Place the palms of your hands on the floor in front of you, and inch them forward as you bend towards them from your hips. Increase the stretch each time you breathe out. Sit back up, change the cross of your legs and repeat. Then stretch each leg out in turn, and bend forward again. Lastly, straighten both legs and bend forward once more, your hands inching forward on the floor as you bend as far as you can without discomfort.

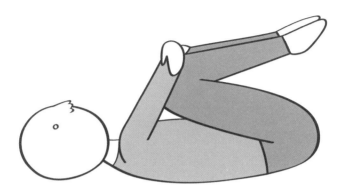

6. Knee hug

Lay down on your back and hug your knees to your chest before resting your legs straight out on the floor. Keep your left leg straight and slowly lift your left foot towards the ceiling, keeping the foot flexed. Repeat with your right leg. Then hug your knees to your chest again, before resting your legs on the floor again.

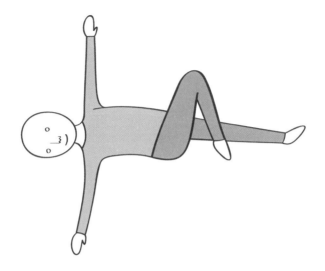

7. Spine twist

Lift your right knee and rest it on the floor on the left side of your body. Stretch your arms straight out on both sides and turn your head to the right. Repeat on the other side. Then rest your legs out straight again, and place your hands by your sides. Stay here and breathe deeply and slowly five times.

#7 DIY acupressure

A traditional Chinese cure for insomnia uses acupressure (needle-free acupuncture) on specific areas of the body. Gently massage these areas to benefit:

• Between your eyebrows, at the top of your nose

• On the inside of your wrist, just off-centre on the opposite side to your pulse

• On the lobes of your ears

• On your soles, just beneath the ball of your foot

• On the top of your feet, between the joints of your big toe and second toe

"Think in the morning.
Act in the noon.
Eat in the evening.
Sleep in the night."

WILLIAM BLAKE
English poet (1757 – 1827)

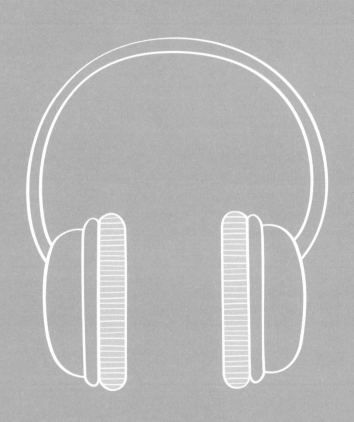

#8 The sleep playlist

During the day, put together a playlist of songs with sleep as their theme. In the evening, turn the lights down low, settle yourself somewhere warm and comfortable and listen to each song in turn.

To get you started, try Good Night by The Beatles, Lullaby by Johannes Brahms and Lazy Head by Alisha's Attic.

"Drag your thoughts away from
your troubles...by the ears,
by the heels, or any other
way you can manage it."

MARK TWAIN
American writer (1835 – 1910)

#9 Out with the old

Having clean bedsheets is the second best thing in life that's free (after cuddles), according to a survey.

The feel and smell of fresh sheets certainly makes your bed more inviting, so peel off the old covers and replace with clean ones at least once per fortnight.

Having a clean and tidy bedroom can also help you feel calmer and more restful, too, so take the time to put away any loose items before you settle under your duvet.

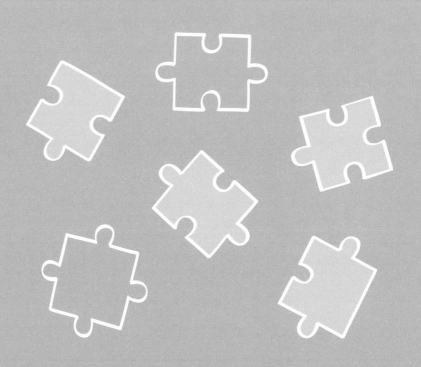

#10 Traditional pastimes

We're so used to being entertained by our digital devices that it's sometimes hard to know what to do without them. Tonight, as part of your wind-down routine, pick a retro activity to try before heading to bed.

For example, you could do a puzzle, fill in a colouring book, try drawing some objects around you, learn to sew or knit, bake your own bread, read a fiction book, have a bath or listen to an audiobook.

Use this part of the day to do things you love and enjoy that you wouldn't otherwise get time for.

#11 Binaural beats

Delivering different sound frequencies to each ear causes your brain to process a completely new frequency, one that would be too quiet to hear through normal audio.

This technique can be used to mimic brainwaves that characterise deep relaxation. Your brain will synchronise to this frequency, helping you to quickly switch mental gears from more active brainwaves.

To benefit, download meditation tracks that use binaural beats and play them through headphones in the evenings.

"You wouldn't worry so much
about what others think of you
if you realised how seldom they do."

ELEANOR ROOSEVELT
Former First Lady of the US (1884 – 1962)

#12 Keep a sleep diary

Professor Jason Ellis, Director of the Northumbria Centre for Sleep Research, recommends keeping a sleep diary.

Each night, note down what you did, ate and drank that day. Write down what time you are getting into bed and how tired you feel. In the morning, add roughly how long it took you to fall asleep, whether you woke during the night and how long you were awake for. Rate how well you slept and how tired you feel now.

After a few days, start to look for patterns. Are you sleeping worse on days when you've had alcohol? Are you sleeping better on days when you've had exercise? Use this information to decide on any changes you need to make.

"A well-spent day brings happy sleep."

LEONARDO DA VINCI
Italian polymath (1452 – 1519)

#13 Stomach massage

De-stress your stomach muscles and organs by using a soft ball as a massage aid for five minutes before going to bed. Use a ball that's about 20 inches in circumference - a child's bouncy ball can work well.

Place the ball on the floor, then position yourself on all fours with the ball gently pushing into your stomach. Rotate over the ball in all directions to loosen any areas of tension, while breathing slowly and deeply into your stomach.

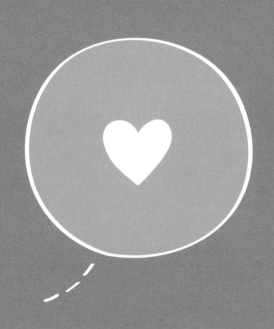

#14 Repeat a mantra

When preparing for bed, psychologist Suzy Reading says to herself, 'There is nothing required of me right now' as many times as necessary for her to relax.

She explains, "Taking time to 'set aside' whatever your body or mind is demanding right now acts like a friend's voice - and is deeply comforting."

#15 Use sleep-inducing scents

Buy an essential oil in a relaxing scent such as lavender, jasmine or sandalwood. Add drops to an oil burner, or dab the scent on the part of your wrist where you can feel your pulse.

#16 Make friends with stress

Health psychologist Kelly McGonigal reports that how we think about the impact of stress affects how our body responds to it. If you believe stress to be harmful, your body has a negative physical reaction to it. If you view stress as an expected part of life, and trust in your ability to cope with whatever life throws at you, your body's response will be much healthier.

Research also shows that connecting with - and caring for - others during challenging times increases our stress resilience, so phone a friend, help a relative out or chat to a loved one.

#17 Begin a tea ritual

Slip on your favourite pyjamas, lower the lights and sip slowly on a herbal tea. Chamomile tea and valerian tea both have proven relaxation qualities, and enjoying them on a regular basis before sleep will help train your brain that it's time to prepare for sleep.

"Live in the moment,
Notice what is happening on purpose,
Choose how you respond to
your experiences,
Rather than being driven by
habitual reactions."

VIDYAMALA BURCH
British mindfulness author and trainer

#18 The joy of journalling

Unlike keeping a diary, journalling is not about recording events. It's about reflecting on your thoughts and feelings and releasing your emotions out from your head and on to paper. All you need is a notebook, pen and somewhere to sit and write before going to bed each night.

Open to a fresh page and start writing, without judgement or censorship. Some prompts to get you started are:

- What are you grateful for?

- What scares and excites you at the moment?

- When have you felt most proud, of yourself and those you care about?

- What kind of things make you laugh uncontrollably?

- What recent moments of joy have you experienced?

- What have been some recent challenges and achievements?

- When have you felt at total peace with yourself and the world?

- What are your hopes and dreams for the future?

"The greatest weapon against stress is our ability to choose one thought over another."

WILLIAM JAMES
American philosopher and psychologist (1842–1910)

#19 Tap it out

Tapping is based on the principles of acupuncture, but thankfully it doesn't require any needles. Practitioner Gary Craig recommends gently tapping your fingertips on different areas of your body in this sequence to feel immediate benefits:

- Top of the head
- Beginning of the eyebrow
- Side of the eye
- Under the eye
- Under the nose
- Chin point
- Beginning of the collarbone
- Under the arm

#20 Apply the rule of five

What worries are on your mind? Will they matter in five days? Five weeks? Five years? If not, perhaps they're not as big an issue as they seem right now.

Use this technique to develop your sense of perspective, so you can step outside of your worries and see them more objectively.

#21 Mindful music

During the day, put together a playlist of the most relaxing, calming tunes you can find. In the evening, dim the lights, sit or lay somewhere comfortable, put on headphones and listen to each song.

Focus your attention on the lyrics, melody and feeling of the music, noticing details that you wouldn't pick up on if it was just playing in the background. Admire the skill and effort that went into creating it, and enjoy listening to the music for its own sake.

"I go to bed early.
My favourite dream
comes on at nine."

EDDIE IZZARD
English comedian, actor & writer

#22 Let the sun go down in your house

You've probably heard of sunrise lamps that gradually wake you up with a brightening light. There are now sunset lamps (or combination lamps), that lose their light intensity over a period of half an hour or so. They tell your body that it's time to go to sleep by mimicking nature's clock-in-the-sky, the sun.

Alternatively, you can mimic this effect with mood lighting. Set up gentle sources of light in the rooms you use in the evenings so you can switch off your main, overhead lightbulbs.

PART III

Calm your mind

You've implemented the Good Sleep Habits and given yourself time to wind down before bed. Now, as you slip under the bedsheets, take one of these techniques with you.

You'll be trying out some peaceful visualisations, changing how you think about sleep and putting into practice a range of practical techniques. They all help to calm and occupy your mind so that you can relax into restful slumber.

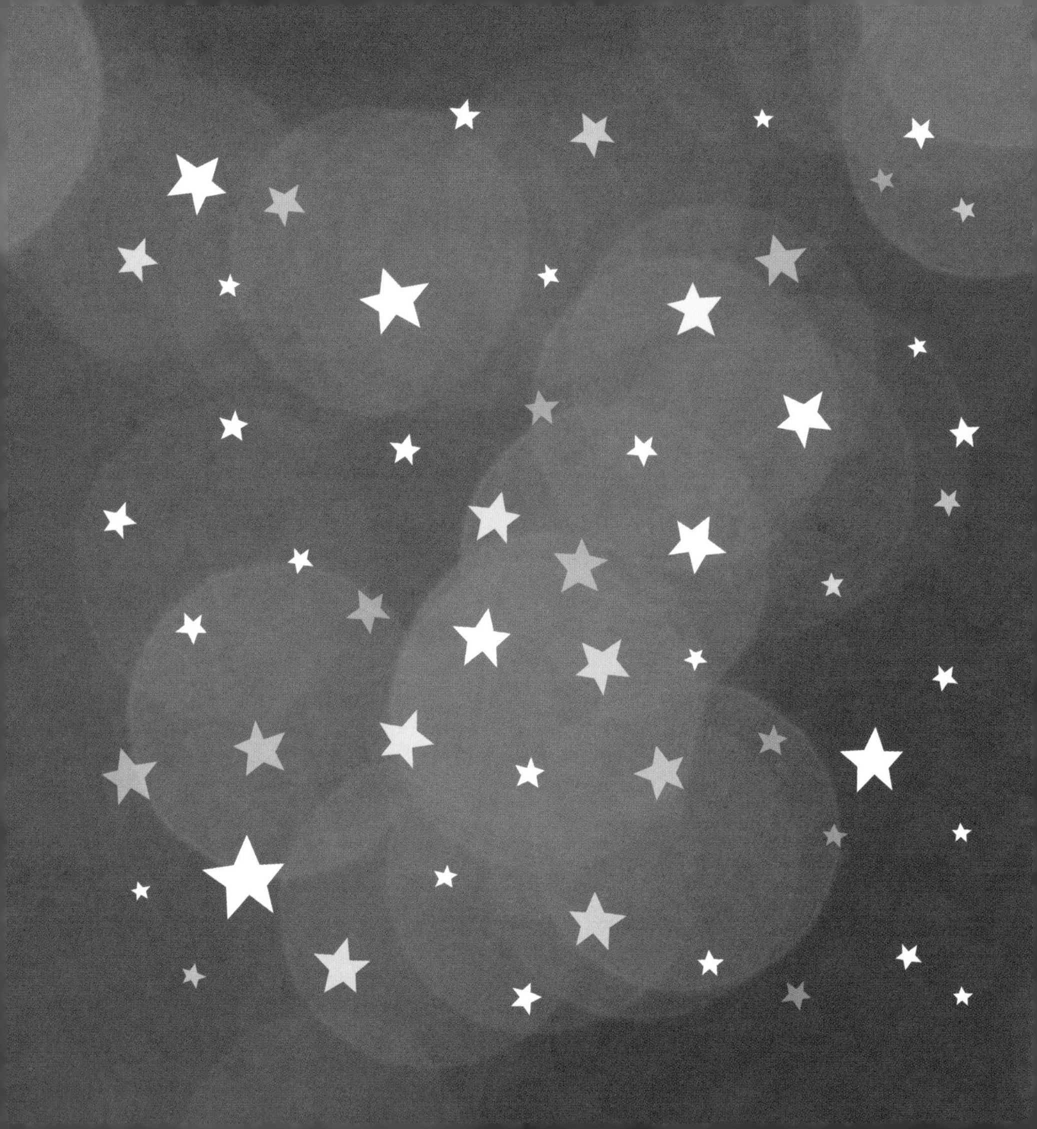

"O bed! O bed! delicious bed!
That heaven upon earth to
the weary head."

THOMAS HOOD
English poet (1799 - 1845)

#1 Do a tension scan

Starting from either your toes or the top of your head, work your way across the length of your body, focusing on each area in turn. Mentally 'scan' that area for tension.

If you find any, relax it, either by contracting and releasing the muscle, or by mentally instructing that body part to relax. Continue through every part, including your eye sockets, tongue, scalp and all of your fingers and toes.

#2 Sleep affirmations

In his book, *Say Goodnight to Insomnia*, Dr Gregg D. Jacobs advocates swapping your negative thoughts about sleep with positive ones. Whenever you have a negative thought about your sleep, choose to replace it with one of these:

- "I always go to sleep sooner or later."

- "My sleep will improve as I learn these new techniques."

- "I am probably sleeping better and for longer than I think I am."

- "I will be able to cope just fine tomorrow, even if I feel tired."

- "I don't need to worry about sleep."

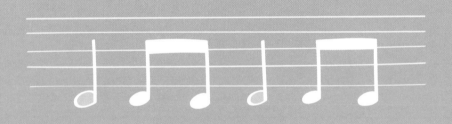

#3 Monotone narrator

In Paul McKenna's book, *I Can Make You Sleep*, he recalls some research shared with him by Dr Win Wenger. Dr Wenger found that when people mentally described the stream of thoughts passing through their mind, they quickly became sleepy.

Once you're in bed, close your eyes and use a slow, monotone internal voice inside your head to narrate whatever you become aware of.

For example, "I can hear the sound of rustling tree leaves outside. Now I can see the row of trees outside my house. Now I remember the smell of pine cones. Now I see a leaf floating in a river." No matter what comes into your head, keep describing it using a calm monotone, like a bored voiceover artist on a tv show.

"A good laugh and a long sleep are the best cures in the doctor's book."

IRISH PROVERB

#4 Summer picnic visualisation

Imagine yourself on a thick, patchwork rug on a large patch of grass, dotted with trees. A traditional wicker basket is propped up on one corner of the rug, now emptied of its delicious contents. The sun is softening from its midday peak, and you lay down, feeling full and satisfied from your picnic feast.

You look to one side and see butterflies lazily spinning from one flower to the next. To your other side, your friend is snoozing, eyes closed and a smile on their face.

In the distance, you can hear children laughing and playing. You have nothing to do for the rest of the afternoon but relax and enjoy being here in this beautiful place.

#5 Change the soundtrack

Got an annoying song stuck on repeat in your head?
Consciously replace it with a more calming, appropriate
one. My go-to song is the Christmas Carol Silent Night.

#6 Nodcasts

The UK's Sleep Council asked 2,000 people which sounds helped them to go to sleep. Among the top answers were birdsong, rain, thunder, waves and wind.

Download audio tracks with these sounds, and play them on repeat while you're in bed.

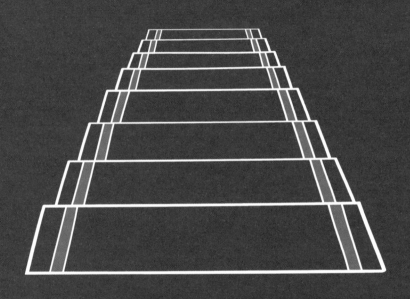

#7 The ten stairs visualisation

Imagine your perfect place, with colours, smells, scenes and decor that feel most safe and welcoming to you. To get to this place, you need to go down ten steps.

Visualise yourself standing at the top of the staircase, feeling calm and positive, looking forward to making your way down. Mentally count down the steps as you slowly take them, imagining your foot gently sinking into each step.

When you arrive, explore the details and sensations of this safe, special place that's unique and perfect for you.

#8 Luxurious sleep

In his book, *Sleep Smarter*, Shawn Stevenson recommends reframing your perception of sleep. Instead of thinking of sleep as something you have to do, start thinking of it as something you get to do.

Consider it to be a treat you can indulge in everyday - a luxury like eating an amazing dessert, enjoying a relaxing massage or something else that you really look forward to.

"Sleep is one of the great pleasures of life."

TWIGGY
English model

#9 The wooden boat visualisation

Imagine yourself in a traditional rowing boat, floating on a large, calm lake. Your friend is oaring lazily, making the boat glide in large, slow figure-of-eight loops across the surface of the water.

You hear the little splashes of water hitting the sides of the craft as the oars sweep inwards. You watch the clouds form shapes and rotate above you as you laze back contentedly.

"For my part, I know nothing with any certainty, but the sight of the stars makes me dream."

VINCENT VAN GOGH
Dutch painter (1853 – 1890)

Z 10
Z 10
Z 10

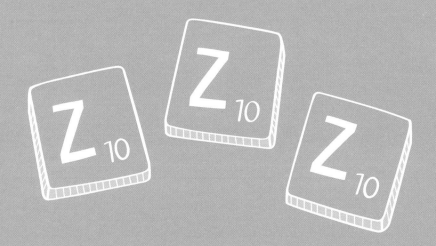

#10 Play sleep-related word games

Think of a positive word that relates to sleep, such as 'peaceful'. Then think of another word, starting with the last letter of the previous one - 'l' in this case, so 'lazy'. Then another - 'yawn', and so on.

#11 Reverse telescope

Keep replaying an event in your head? Try this to get perspective on your worries. Visualise the scene again, but this time start to zoom out from your initial perspective.

See the room from above, then the building and the local area. Keep zooming out - see the region, the country and eventually the planet. Mentally watch the planet turning slowly on its axis, amid the weather, the moon and stars.

#12 Sun, sea and sand

Picture yourself reclining on a deckchair under a palm tree, somewhere in the Maldives or Caribbean. You've just had a delicious lunch with a loved one at the beachside restaurant. Now you have nothing to do but lie back and relax.

Imagine the sweep and retreat of the calm sea, matching the flow of your breath. Feel the warmth of the sun on your skin, smell the salty tang of the sea air and watch the white sailboats glide elegantly from one end of the bay to the other.

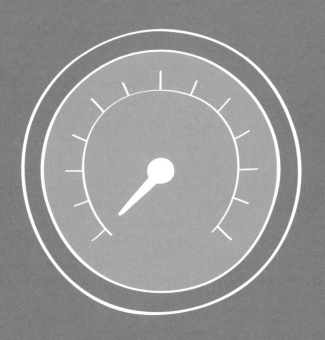

#13 Slow down your breathing

The 4-7-8 technique was pioneered by Dr Andrew Weil, a holistic health doctor. First, lightly rest your tongue against the tissue behind your top front teeth. Then:

1. Breathe in through your nose for four seconds
2. Hold your breath for seven seconds
3. Exhale through your mouth for eight seconds
4. Repeat

"If you can't sleep, then get
up and do something instead
of lying there worrying.
It's the worrying that gets you,
not the lack of sleep."

DALE CARNEGIE
American writer & self improvement trainer (1888 – 1955)

#14 Change your focus

In her book, *The Effortless Sleep Method*, Sasha Stephens advises that if you are lying in bed but no longer feeling sleepy, get up and do something else, such as reading a book, piecing together a puzzle or doing the ironing. The intention is to ensure a healthy association between being in your bed and feeling sleepy.

Decide in advance what it is you will do, so that you go to bed knowing that if you sleep, great, but if not, you'll get up and do whatever activity you have picked instead.

#15 Worrying about something?

Can you do something about the source of your worry?
If yes, great. Do it or write down a reminder for the morning.

If you can't do anything about it, then there's no point
worrying. Make peace with uncertainty.

#16 Change your tone

In Paul McKenna's book, *I Can Make You Sleep*, he suggests you bring to mind one of your beliefs about your inability to sleep. Mentally state the the belief now, and notice whereabouts the voice in your head is located.

Repeat the phrase again, but move the voice so it seems further away in the distance. Notice what the tone of your internal voice is.

Repeat the belief again, and this time change the tone of your internal voice so it becomes calm and drowsy.

Next, repeat the phrase with a yawn between each word. Do this whenever an unhelpful thought comes to mind.

"There have been plenty of nights where you have actually slept quite well... From this moment, commit to focusing only on all that is good about your sleeping. Start telling a new story."

SASHA STEPHENS
Author of The Effortless Sleep Method

"Mindfulness is not designed to get you to sleep, but rather increases your willingness to experience the discomfort associated with not sleeping. When you accept what shows up in the middle of the night, you are less likely to react emotionally and more likely to sleep in the long run."

DR GUY MEADOWS
Founder of the Sleep School and author of The Sleep Book

#17 Nighttime mindfulness

In *The Sleep Book*, Dr Guy Meadows advises noticing and accepting what you are thinking and feeling.

First, notice the feel of your mattress below you. Then scan your body for sensations or urges, starting from your toes and gradually sweeping upwards.

Welcome and accept whatever you notice, whether it's your beating heart, an urge to move or a worrying thought. Don't judge it, or try to change it. Just notice and accept its existence peacefully.

#18 Find your smile

If you notice yourself frowning, then smile, even if you're in bed. It releases the tensed facial muscles and makes you feel instantly better, whether or not it's sincere.

#19 The biggest bed visualisation

Imagine you are lying on the biggest bed in the world. It's so big that you can't see the edges of it, nor the walls of the room that's holding it. The sheets and duvet are pure white, and the pillows are plentiful.

The bed is the most comfortable you have ever experienced, and you lie there, delighted to have the vast space of it to yourself. There is nothing for you to do but enjoy being in this bed, with as much room as you desire to stretch, move and relax in.

#20 Label your thoughts

In *The Sleep Book*, Dr Guy Meadows recommends identifying common thoughts you have about sleep and giving them a label.

For example, 'If I don't sleep tonight I won't be able to cope tomorrow' becomes 'coping' and 'It's not fair, why can they sleep and I can't?' becomes 'jealousy'.

Then, when the thought occurs, welcome it. Mentally say 'Welcome back, coping' or 'Good to see you again, jealousy'. Thank your mind for bringing up the thought. Repeat the thought in a funny voice, or sing a song to it.

You can also apply this technique to your emotions. Identify them, describe them, locate their whereabouts in your body. What are they doing? What do they look and feel like? Imagine them as over-the-top characters on a theatre stage.

The goal is to remove the power of the thought or emotion by seeing it and responding to it in a new way.

#21 You've got a friend in you

Feeling frustrated, angry or stressed? Imagine explaining to a close friend how you feel right now. What would they say to you? Start saying that to yourself, using the same tone of voice as your friend would.

"It ain't as bad as you think.
It will look better in the morning."

COLIN POWELL
American statesman & retired army general

#22 The thought locker

Professor Colin Espie, Founder and CEO of The Sleepio program, suggests imagining a glass box attached to the wall above your bed. Whenever a worry comes to mind, mentally open the lid and put the thought inside the box.

If the worry returns to your thoughts, remind yourself that it's safely in the locker and you will deal with it in the morning.

#23 Do nothing

In *The Effortless Sleep Method*, Sasha Stephens shares her favourite relaxation technique.

She says, "Lie down, turn out the light and do nothing. It is important not to 'try' to do nothing. Do not avoid thinking about sleep, nor try to think about sleep... If thoughts arise, let them. Don't engage with them, or try to stop them... Just 'do' nothing at all."

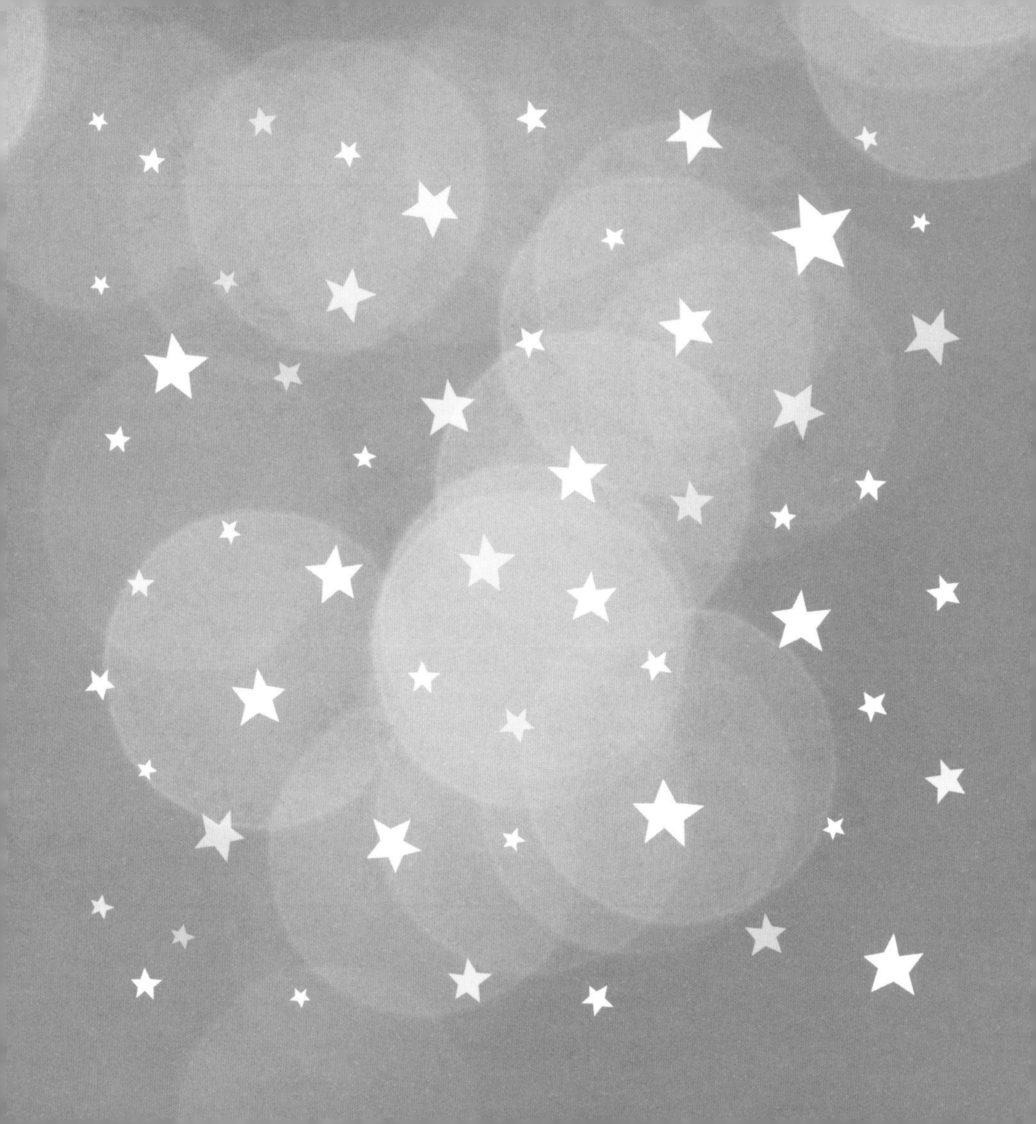

"God grant me the serenity to accept the things I cannot change; courage to change the things I can; and wisdom to know the difference."

REINHOLD NIEBUHR
American theologian (1892–1971)

#24 A novel retreat visualisation

Think of two lovable characters from the world of fiction. They decide to take a day off from their usual adventures in order to relax and enjoy each other's company.

Use your imagination to mentally watch the day unfold. Where do they go? What do they talk about? Does romance blossom?

#25 Change your sleep beliefs

In *This Book Will Make You Sleep*, Dr Jessamy Hibberd and Jo Usmar recommend changing your beliefs about sleep. Neutralise your worries by accepting the following (true) statements about sleep:

- I will fall asleep eventually

- I do sleep more than I realise

- I will function just fine tomorrow and will cope even if I feel a little tired

- My body can handle periods of sleeplessness

- How I feel in the morning won't dictate my day

If you find yourself thinking thoughts that contradict any of the above five statements, correct yourself with the truth, using a warm, kind and positive mental voice to do so.

"We are such stuff as
dreams are made on;
and our little life is
rounded with a sleep."

WILLIAM SHAKESPEARE
English poet, playwright & actor (1564 – 1616)

#26 Golden glow visualisation

In his book *Calm*, author Michael Acton Smith suggests imagining a golden light above you. Visualise its warmth gradually starting to fill every cell of your body with a sense of peace, from your head to your toes.

Feel your weight begin to slowly lighten, then imagine yourself lifting from the ground and floating towards the golden glow, through the sky and clouds. Notice how peaceful you feel.

#27 The snowstorm visualisation

Imagine you are walking through thick snow, with fresh snowflakes swirling to the ground around you. The snow crunches beneath your boots as you take each step.

The falling snow is becoming thicker and thicker, but you keep your eyes focused on the glowing dome of your igloo, which is now only a few metres away. You slide in through the entrance on your stomach, then seal it behind you by rolling a slab of ice in front of it.

The wind and the noise is silenced immediately and the candle lighting the interior flickers more gently. Your bed is a makeshift pile of furs and fabrics and you gratefully settle yourself into it, feeling safe, cosy and protected from the elements. Your body starts to warm up and feels deeply relaxed.

#28 Banish worries from your mental movie set

If an unwanted thought comes to mind, imagine it morphing into a cartoon version of itself. Then picture your finger and thumb flicking it away with a firm 'no'. This is your movie and you are the director.

#29 That sinking feeling

Imagine your body getting heavier each time you slowly breathe out. Feel your weight sinking into the mattress as the air leaves your body.

Focus on the growing sensation of heaviness across each limb and muscle. Start to feel so heavy that moving any part of your body becomes impossible.

"Laughter and tears are both responses to frustration and exhaustion. I myself prefer to laugh, since there is less cleaning up to do afterward."

KURT VONNEGUT
American writer (1922 – 2007)

#30 Tidal breaths

Breathe deeply into your stomach, feeling it gradually expand. Imagine your inhalation washing over your mind like a wave on the seashore. Feel it rinse away your cares, thoughts and worries.

Exhale slowly. Imagine the wave receding and sweeping away all your mental debris, like grains of sand carried back to the sea. Repeat.

"Normal sleepers are willing to relax and be quietly wakeful in the pre-sleep phase. They aren't trying to force sleep upon themselves, but are happy to ride along with it, knowing that even if they don't sleep, they are still getting some much-needed rest."

DR GUY MEADOWS

Founder of the Sleep School and author of The Sleep Book

#31 Thought blocking

Can't stop thinking about a worry? In *This Book Will Make You Sleep*, Dr Jessamy Hibberd and Jo Usmar suggest picking a word that is completely neutral for you - for example, 'one' or 'the' - and mentally repeating it every two or three seconds.

It's hard to think about two things at once, so this technique blocks out the unwanted thought.

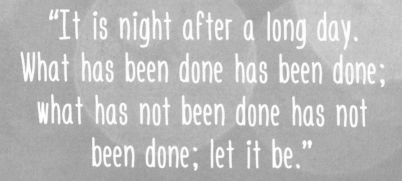

"It is night after a long day. What has been done has been done; what has not been done has not been done; let it be."

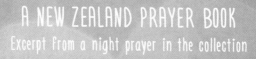

A NEW ZEALAND PRAYER BOOK

Excerpt from a night prayer in the collection

#32 Have a safety thought

In her book, *The Effortless Sleep Method*, Sasha Stephens recommends picking "a comfortable and encouraging fact about your sleep" to bring you hope when you're in bed.

For example, 'I slept through worries like this before and I can do it again' or 'I slept in a different bed before so I know I can sleep in this one' or 'I coped before after not sleeping very much so it doesn't matter whether or not I sleep'. Then get into bed feeling good about that fact and relaxing into it as you lie down.

"Nothing in life is quite as important as you think it is while you're thinking about it."

DANIEL KAHNEMAN

Israeli-American psychologist and behavioural economist

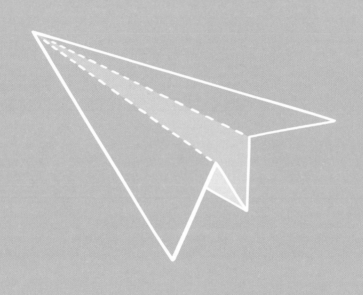

#33 Watch your worries fly away

Every time a worry comes to mind, imagine writing it on a piece of paper. Mentally fold the paper into a small square or an origami shape and leave it on the bedroom windowsill. Picture a gentle breeze lifting it up from the sill and carrying it far away.

#34 Challenge your beliefs

In *This Book Will Make You Sleep*, authors Dr Jessamy Hibberd and Jo Usmar suggest challenging your thoughts and beliefs about sleep.

For example, if you think 'I'm not going to be able to sleep tonight', actively look for proof that this statement is false. Remember previous times when you thought that you wouldn't sleep well, but actually, you slept fine.

This will help you accept that your thoughts and beliefs are just thoughts and beliefs - not facts.

"Thoughts aren't facts so don't take them seriously."

RUBY WAX

British / American actress & mental health campaigner

#35 Childhood home visualisation

Bring to mind your childhood home. Picture yourself wandering around it, exploring each room in turn and trying to remember as many details as you can.

What was the decoration, furniture and atmosphere in each room? Which rooms did you spend most time in, and what did you do in them? Which were your favourite rooms and why?

#36 Remember a favourite novel

Think of a book you enjoyed, then mentally retrace what happened. How did the story start? What were the characters like? How did they change and develop by the end of the book?

Bring to mind as much detail as you can, and visualise the characters, their surroundings and the events of the book vividly.

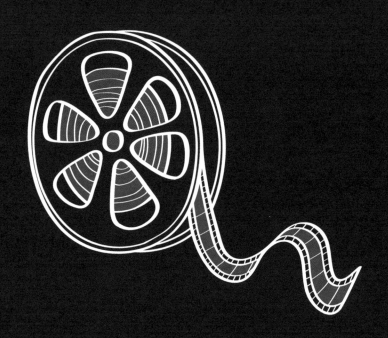

#37 Your perfect day visualisation

You're in a cinema from the 1970s. You've got the screening room to yourself and you're sitting on a plush, red chair. The velvet armrests feel soft under your elbows. The screen flickers to life and the house lights fade.

The words 'Your perfect day' form on-screen in a curvy, handwritten font. The projector ticks softly from somewhere behind you as the spool winds forward.

Vividly imagine the rest of the film in sensory detail, picturing your ideal morning, afternoon and evening. Play your favourite moments in slow motion, with suitably soft and uplifting music to accompany those scenes.

"My life has been filled with terrible misfortune, most of which never happened."

MICHEL DE MONTAIGNE
French philosopher, writer and politican (1533-1592)

#38 Retrace your thoughts

Follow your train of thought backwards, remembering how each one led to the next. Start with your current thought, then try to recall the thought that prompted it, then the one before that.

Keep going back as far as you can, and repeat the process whenever you notice that you're thinking about something again.

#39 Re-live your day

Zen guru Leo Babauta recommends relaxing by remembering the details of your day:

"...close your eyes, and visualize what you did first thing today. That might be opening your eyes and getting out of bed. Then visualize the second thing you did — let's say you peed and washed your face, or drank a glass of water... Visualize these tiny steps in detail. I never get past the first hour before I'm asleep."

"Everything has its wonders,
even darkness and silence, and
I learn whatever state I may
be in, therein to be content."

HELEN KELLER
American author and activist (1880 – 1968)

#40 Relax like a yogi

One of the relaxation techniques used in yoga is guiding your attention around each part of your body.

For example, start with the tips of your fingers on one hand. Focus on them intently. Then let that attention travel slowly up your arms, into your chest and down through your stomach, leg and toes. Return up and over the other half of your body.

#41 Feel the feelings

Lester Levenson, creator of the Sedona Method, believes that allowing ourselves to experience our emotions, then release them, can enable easier, better sleep.

So identify your emotions about sleep (such as fear of not sleeping) or your feelings about today or tomorrow. Feel the feeling, immerse yourself in it. Then, make a decision to let that feeling go. Release it. Allow it to leave now, just as you allowed yourself to feel it.

"I set out a series of problems
for myself and I write them
down, and when I'm sleeping,
my mind solves the problems.
When I wake up in the morning,
I have more clarity on the issue."

WYNTON MARSALIS
American jazz musician

#42 Through the woods visualisation

Visualise yourself walking through woodland, with age-old trees around you and dappled sunlight freckling the path in front of you. The air is warm and still, with occasional welcome breezes.

You follow the path and come to a wooden bridge over a stream. You stop to admire the water, and spot red-gold fish gliding to and fro under the surface. You continue, coming to the edge of the woods just as a dark cloud approaches. You walk towards a wood-built cabin ahead of you, increasing your pace to a jog as the first drops of rain splash onto the grass around you.

You reach the cabin at the very second that the rain turns to a downpour, and let yourself in gratefully. You drop your tired body into a rocking chair, tilt back your head and rest your eyes as you listen to the raindrops against the window.

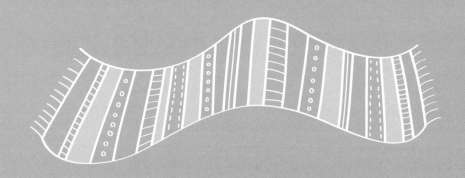

#43 The magic carpet visualisation

Imagine you're safely tucked into your sleeping bag on a big, magic carpet. The carpet gently rises from the ground, the windows of your room automatically open and you are transported out to the clear, cool night.

Imagine the stars in their formations above you, and the streetlights and occasional vehicle travelling around your village, town or city below you. You snuggle deeper into your sleeping bag, enjoying the warmth it provides.

The gentle movements of the carpet make you relax, and you struggle to keep your eyes open as you tour your neighbourhood from this unique viewpoint.

#44 Childhood memory

Recall a happy moment from your childhood. Picture the scene, the smells, the atmosphere. Feel as though the clock has rewound and you are now back there. Relive the moment, imagining any details you've forgotten.

"What a magical thing is the bed, and what a vulnerable, innocent creature is the sleeping human – the human who never looks more truthful or pitiful or benign; the curled-up, childlike dreaming soul who has for a few hours become an angel adrift."

MICHAEL LEUNIG
Australian artist & cartoonist

#45 In with the good, out with the bad

Picture tension and worries leaving your body with each out-breath. Imagine calm and relaxation entering your body with each in-breath.

#46 Retrain your responses

Do you sometimes jerk awake, either after a falling sensation or just as you're about to drift off?

In *The Sleep Book*, Dr Guy Meadows teaches readers to give that reaction a name, and acknowledge it playfully when it next happens. Don't otherwise worry about it or react to it.

Your new, calmer response will train your brain that no threat exists and that it's ok to stay relaxed and sleepy, even when you jerk awake.

"Not minding about whether you sleep is probably the one single most important (and difficult) change in attitude that you can make... When you don't care whether you will sleep or not, all pressure is gone and sleep comes so much more easily..."

SASHA STEPHENS
Author of The Effortless Sleep Method

#47 Tired friends

In Paul McKenna's book, *I Can Make You Sleep*, he suggests remembering a time when you felt very tired, then visualising yourself surrounded by friends who are just as tired as you.

Picture one of them yawning, then another and another. Watch them struggling and failing to keep their eyes open, and let youself yawn and close your eyes, too.

Notice a calm, warm feeling spreading through and around you. If your mind drifts, bring it back to imagining yourself looking around the circle of tired, sleepy faces.

"The English expression 'to fall asleep' is apt because the transition between waking and sleeping is a gradual drop from one state of being into another: a giving up of full self-consciousness for unconsciousness or for the altered consciousness of dreams."

SIRI HUSTVEDT
American author

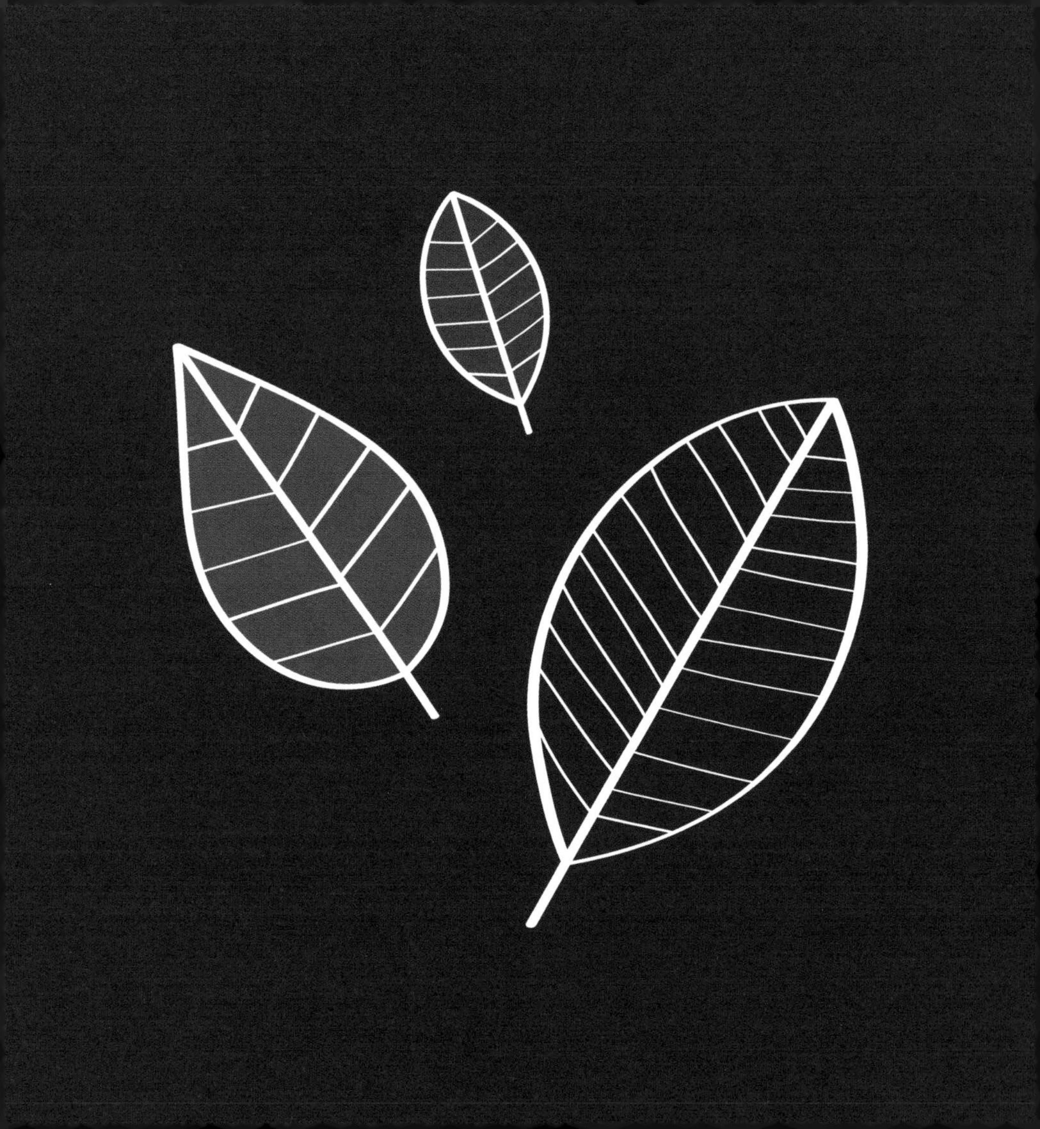

#48 Autumn leaves visualisation

Imagine a tree in the Autumn, with hundreds of burnished red, gold and brown leaves. One by one, each leaf falls loose and spins slowly to the soft grass beneath.

Visualise flocks of birds flying overhead to warmer climates, squirrels burying food for winter snacks and chubby hedgehogs preparing their nests for hibernation.

Imagine the air becoming cooler and the leaves continuing to drop, as you snuggle gratefully into the safe, warm cocoon of your duvet.

"It is a common experience that a problem difficult at night is resolved in the morning after the committee of sleep has worked on it."

JOHN STEINBECK
American author (1902 – 1968)

#49 Change the ending

Bad dream? Professor Jason Ellis, Director of the Northumbria Centre for Sleep Research, advises that you write it down while it's still vivid. Then write down how you would have liked to change your dream.

For example, if you dreamt you were being chased, write down that you had wings and soared away from your pursuers, or that the pursuers were friends who were trying to keep up with you as you surged to the finish line of a marathon. This puts you back in control, and helps you reframe your dream in a more positive way.

#50 Bring in a new perspective

In his book, *Say Goodnight to Insomnia*, Dr Gregg D. Jacobs suggests challenging negative thoughts by asking yourself questions such as:

- Is this thought really true?
- Am I overemphasising a negative aspect of the situation?
- What is the worst thing that will happen?
- Is there another way to look at this situation?
- What difference will this make next week, month or year?

#51 Clifftop retreat visualisation

Imagine that you've been travelling for some time, and have finally arrived at your destination.

It's a beautiful stone building on a clifftop, overlooking the sparkling blue-green sea in the distance. The back doors are set wide open to let the air circulate, and the voile curtains lift and play in the breeze.

Behind you, a large white bed beckons, and your body aches to lie upon it. First, though you look out to sea, savouring the view and the joy of having finally arrived.

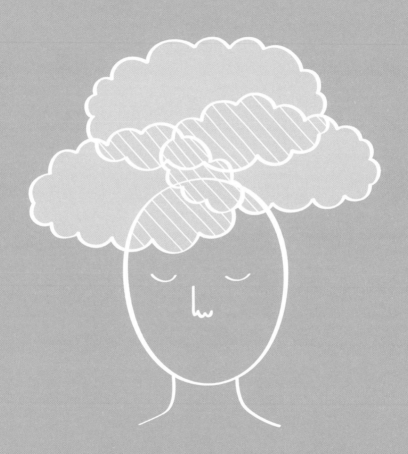

#52 You are not your thoughts

Distance yourself from your thinking.

Watch your thoughts form, fade and pass like waves on a beach or clouds in the sky. Don't judge or interact with them, just let them pass.

"Sleep is the best meditation."

DALAI LAMA
Tibetan Buddhist monk

#53 Slow counting

Count backwards, slowly, from 250 to 1. If your mind wanders off, gently bring it back to the last number you remember counting. Then continue. 250... 249... 248...

#54 Become the breath

In her book, *The Effortless Sleep Method*, Sasha Stephens recommends going one step further than focusing on your breathing. She says, "Try shifting your focus from watching the breath to being the breath". Repeat to yourself, 'I am the breath' and feel your sense of self merging with your inhalations and exhalations.

In the same way, you can inhabit your feelings and emotions about sleep. Do you feel scared that you won't sleep? Feel the fear, welcome the fear, then become the fear. Say to yourself, 'I am the fear'. This reveals the fear to be nothing more than a perception, an idea. It disappears and neutralises once you are no longer scared of it.

"The only thing that I'm obsessed with is sleeping, and actually, it is more than an obsession, it is a pleasure."

CHRISTIAN BALE
British actor

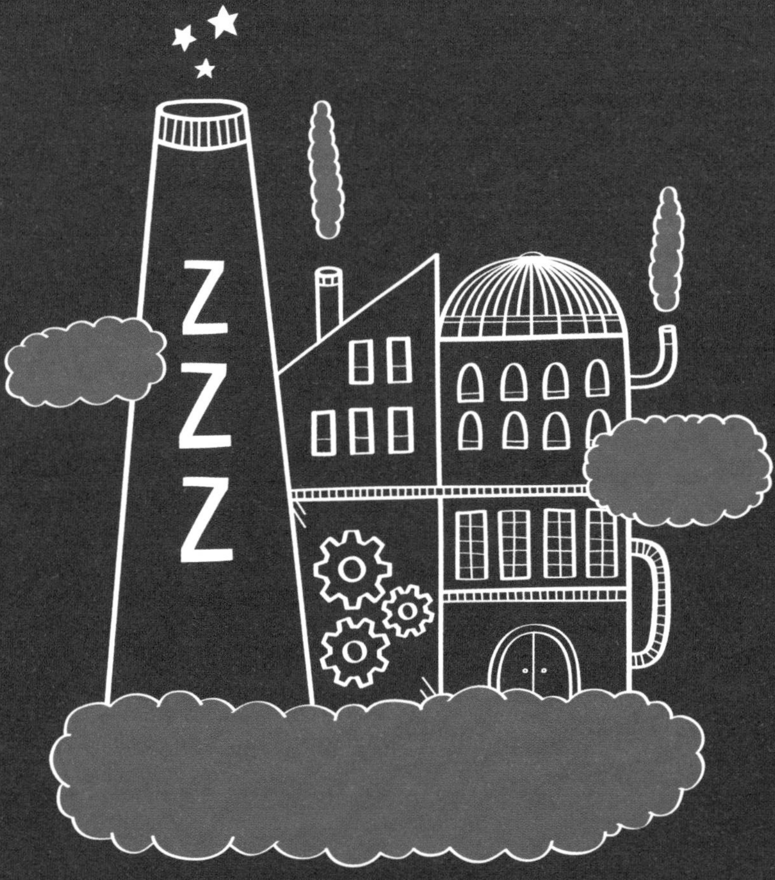
ZZZ

#55 The dream factory visualisation

Picture yourself walking across the soft, candyfloss surface of a cloud, towards a building unlike any you've ever seen before. This is where peaceful dreams are made before they are sent to the dreamer.

You walk through double-height oak doors and are greeted by a tour guide. Your guide takes you into the first room, where you see kittens playing with cotton wool balls, ready to charm and delight animal-lovers.

In the next room, blue-green feathers are being sewn into wings, for the people who dream of taking to the sky each night. Imagine the details of these rooms and many more as you explore the estate fully.

What's in the rooms where your favourite dreams are made?

"Many things – such as loving, going to sleep, or behaving unaffectedly – are done worst when we try hardest to do them."

C.S. LEWIS
English novelist (18989 – 1963)

#56 Tense and relax

Focus on each part of your body in turn - your toes, feet, ankles, legs, bum, stomach, back, neck, shoulders, arms, hands and even your tongue. Tense the muscles in that body part, hold the tension for five seconds, then relax and move to the next one.

Think of each part of your body as being 'put to sleep' by tensing and relaxing it, and then try not to move that part again.

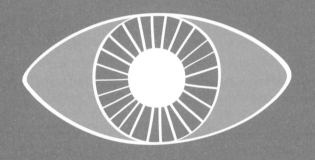

#57 Try not to go to sleep

Instead of aiming to fall asleep, focus on staying awake. This relieves the pressure of trying to make yourself do something that can't be forced.

Keep your eyes open and make a decision to not drift off. Decide to just relax instead, while silently repeating your mantra over and over again: "I will not fall asleep".

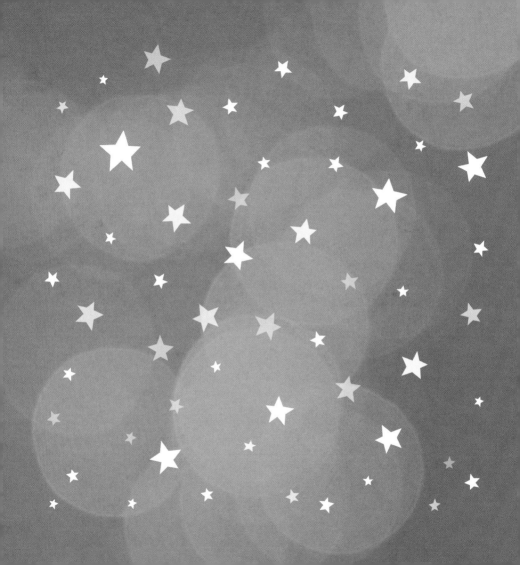

"...and so to bed."

SAMUEL PEPYS
English navy administrator, MP & diarist (1633 - 1703)

REFERENCES

Techniques and visualisations not referenced below are from multiple sources or are the author's own.

Part I

The Good Sleep Habits are combined from multiple printed and online resources, as well as the author's own experience.

Part II

#1 Blue: the sleep hue | https://www.travelodge.co.uk/press-centre/press-releases/SECRET-GOOD-NIGHT'S-SLUMBER-SLEEP-BLUE-BEDROOM

#3 A time to worry; a time to rest | Butler, Gillian and Hope, Tony (2007), Managing Your Mind: The Mental Fitness Guide, Second Edition, USA: OUP

#6 Stretch and relax with yoga | Khalsa, SBS; 2004; Treatment of chronic insomnia with yoga: a preliminary study with sleep-wake diaries; published in Applied Psychophysiology and Biofeedback journal | Stiles, Tara (2010), Slim, Calm, Sexy Yoga, Trade Edition, USA: Rodale Inc | Grime, Louise (2008), 15-Minute Gentle Yoga, London: Dorling Kindersley

#7 DIY acupressure | https://www.acupuncture.org.uk/a-to-z-of-conditions/a-to-z-of-conditions/1283-insomnia.html

#9 Out with the old | http://www.dailymail.co.uk/news/article-2515436/The-best-things-life-free-How-cuddles-country-walks-saying-I-love-everyday-pleasures.html

#11 Binaural beats | https://sleephabits.net/binaural-beats?sfa

#12 Keep a sleep diary | Professor Jason Ellis's sleep diary technique was published in the Daily Mail on 11 February 2017

#13 Stomach massage | Called the 'gut smash', this technique is endorsed by fitness and yoga coach Jill Miller to help relax the stomach area and ease back pain. A number of Jill's fans who have put the technique into practice report also benefitting from improved sleep, including less time to fall asleep and increased sleep quality. Read more here: http://www.crossfitsouthbay.com/holiday-gut-smash/ and here: https://jordansmutscom/2015/09/07/why-gut-smashing-may-be-the-most-beneficial-thing-ive-ever-done/

#14 Repeat a mantra | Psychologist Suzy Reading's mantra technique was published in the November 2016 edition of Psychologies Magazine.

#15 Use sleep-inducing scents | Acton Smith, Michael (2015), Calm, First Edition, UK: Penguin Books

#16 Make friends with stress | https://www.ted.com/talks/kelly_mcgonigal_how_to_make_stress_your_friend

#18 The joy of journalling | Acton Smith, Michael (2015), Calm, First Edition, UK: Penguin Books

#19 Tap it out | http://www.emofree.com/eft-tutorial/tapping-basics/how-to-do-eft.html

Part III

Visualisations | Visualising a relaxing scene helps people fall asleep more quickly, according to research by Oxford University. Conversely, counting sheep made participants in the 2002 study take longer to fall asleep. The findings were discussed in New Scientist magazine. Read more here: www.newscientist.com/article/dn1831-sleep-scientists-discount-sheep/

#2 Sleep affirmations | Jacobs, Gregg (2009), Say Goodnight to Insomnia, London: Rodale/Pan Macmillan

#3 Monotone narrator | McKenna, Paul (2009), I Can Make You Sleep, Fifth edition, London: Bartum Press

#6 Nodcasts | http://www.sleepcouncil.org.uk/nodcasts/

#8 Luxurious sleep | Stevenson, Shawn (2016), Sleep Smarter, UK: Hay House

#13 Slow down your breathing | https://www.drweil.com/videos-features/videos/the-4-7-8-breath-health-benefits-demonstration/

#14 Change your focus | Stephens, Sasha (2010), The Effortless Sleep Method, First Edition, England: Self-Published

#16 Change your tone | McKenna, Paul (2009), I Can Make You Sleep, Fifth edition, London: Bartum Press

#17 Nighttime mindfulness | Meadows, Guy (2014), The Sleep Book, First Edition, Great Britain: Orion

#20 Label your thoughts | Meadows, Guy (2014), The Sleep Book, First Edition, Great Britain: Orion

#22 The thought locker | https://www.sleepio.com/articles/racing-mind/the-thought-locker/

#23 Do nothing | Stephens, Sasha (2010), The Effortless Sleep Method, First Edition, England: Self-Published

#25 Change your sleep beliefs | Hibberd, J. & Usmar, J. (2014), This Book Will Make You Sleep, First Edition, London: Quercus

#26 Golden glow visualisation | Acton Smith, Michael (2015), Calm, First Edition, UK: Penguin Books

#31 Thought blocking | Hibberd, Jessamy & Usmar, Jo (2014), This Book Will Make You Sleep, First Edition, London: Quercus

#32 Have a safety thought | Stephens, Sasha (2010), The Effortless Sleep Method, First Edition, England: Self-Published

#33 Watch your worries fly away | Butler, Gillian and Hope, Tony (2007), Managing Your Mind: The Mental Fitness Guide, Second Edition, USA: OUP

#34 Challenge your beliefs | Hibberd, Jessamy & Usmar, Jo (2014), This Book Will Make You Sleep, First Edition, London: Quercus

#39 Re-live your day | https://zenhabits.net/rockabye/

#41 Feel the feelings | http://www.sedona.com/sleep-and-energy.asp

#46 Retrain your responses | Meadows, Guy (2014), The Sleep Book, First Edition, Great Britain: Orion

#47 Tired friends | McKenna, Paul (2009), I Can Make You Sleep, Fifth edition, London: Bartum Press

#49 Change the ending | Professor Jason Ellis's dream monitoring technique was published in the Daily Mail on 11 February 2017

#50 Bring in a new perspective | Jacobs, Gregg (2009), Say Goodnight to Insomnia, London: Rodale/Pan Macmillan

#52 You are not your thoughts | https://www.ncbi.nlm.nih.gov/pmc/articles/PMC3466342/

#54 Become the breath | Stephens, Sasha (2010), The Effortless Sleep Method, First Edition, England: Self-Published

#56 Tense and relax | Jacobson, E. (1938). Progressive relaxation. Chicago: University of Chicago Press

#57 Try not to go to sleep | Researchers have found that trying to sleep results in performance anxiety, leading to ongoing preoccupation with sleep. One technique to overcome this is Paradoxical Intention Therapy, where you convince yourself you don't care whether or not you sleep because you know you'll fall asleep when you're ready. Read more: Kierlin, L (November 2008). "Sleeping without a pill: nonpharmacologic treatments for insomnia.", Journal of Psychiatric Practice, 14 (6): 403–7

CREDITS

An extra special thank you to:

Alex Lawrence and Gavin O'Brien

Claire Carpenter, Patricia Margaret Taylor, Kathy Dugdale, Christine De Oliveira and Heather Turner

Doug Wellstead and Joyce Wellstead

Jon Wellstead, Eliza Chapman and Mary Rosenna Jones

Lisa Bowen, Carla Dean, Kalam Abul, Richard Boon, Oscar Balladon and Helen Greener

Melody Cohen, Mary Godfrey, Scott Cohen, Charles Tarver White and April Jimenez

Michael Barnstijn

Robyn Roscoe and friends

Sophie Bouilland-Martel, Benjamin Bouilland, Frippon-chat, My Treca HySensation and Vaitéa Martel

Aaron Jamieson

Aarti Rayrella

Adrian Azurin

AJF

Alex

Allan Purkaer

Amy Wilson and
Gemma Peel

Anders F. Årdal

Anders Hovden

Andreas Schubert

Andrey

Ann Noren

Anne Færch Jørgensen

Anonymous

Anonymous

Anonymous

Anonymous

Anthony Carpenter and
Absa-Reena Tasaddiq

Anya Piper and Sarah Rae

Armin J. Salazar

Arvin G. M. and
Czarina Kareel Briones

Baran Ayguler

Benjamin Ball

Billy Anders

Binh Nguyen

BoFiS

Brett A Johnson

Brian Irwin and
Christine DeAngelis

Brooklynn Thomas

Bruce LeCompte

Bryan - MaryLouise
and Jack's Dad

Bryan Pelley

C.M.C.

Cara Gillespie

Ceri Pritchard

Chandra Jessee
and Lorelei Ashe

Chris Niewiarowski

Chris Trimble

Christine Hansen

Claire Nichol

Claire Willers

Clelia Allen

Clément Haenen

Craig McCoy

Cstylinn

Danny Kay Duod

Darryl Brown
and Amy Burke

David and Louise Anderson

Dave Marshall

Deborah Ruth
Goldman Grubman

Denise Eicher
and Kevin Eicher

Dj Padzensky and
Melissa Padzensky

Dominic Ede

Doraleen Smith

Doug Morton

Dr AM Duke

Drew Carpenter

Elena Costales

Elisa Perez

Elisa Lamont

Emma Jane Todd

Eric Damon Waters

Eugene Greenwood

Florian A.

Frahmy on Kangaroo Island

Francesco Ferrari from Verona (Italy)

Francis Siciliano

Gregory S. Bendelius

Gene Harlow

Geoff Snailham

Ghani Raines

Glenn McMath

Greta Zabulyte

Haley

Have a good kip Louisa Moore and pleasant slumbers Linsay Halladay

Heather Addley

Ivan Eissler

Jack Sidaway and Amy Wilding

James Tyler

Jason E Johnston

Jeffrey Eden, Jillian Stearman and Wyatt Eden

Jeff Lewis

Jenny Cole

Jessica Abel

Jherek Rees

Jims

Jin-Kyung Kim

Joey Nguyen

Johanna, Monika and Hans

John A Freeman
- Florida, USA

Jonathan Pallie

Josh Grocott
(BA, MA, PANDA)

Joshua Hodson

Juanfe

Judi Plater

KR

Kate Scott

Katherine Delzell

Katherine Healey

Katy Ratcliffe

Kate Izell

Kendra Waier and
Kassandra Behymer

Kick Mcstarter

Kimberley Timmings

Kirk Braggs

Kirsti Tomlin

Kit Sleepy Lammers

Kourtney DeBoer

Kylu and Kochamczu

Laird Popkin and
Juliette Hartel

Lily Gantchev

Lisa Price

Liz

Lucy Rawkins

Marc Stewart

Maria Stenfelt

Martin Lutz Carlsson

Matthew Alexander Hanna

Mattias Petter Johansson

Max Ocklind

Melvin Wilson Jr.

Meredith Davis
and Bryan Christy

Mike Bundt

Mike Burke

Mike McKerrow

Miche Connor

Michel Verstraeten

Michela Pinner

Nadine Czaika

Nathaniel Hinkel

Nicholas Pinter

Nina Frey

Odin Elijah Plater

Ong Jia Min

Oscar Arenas Larios

Patrick Cantwell

Patrik Spathon

Prelou

Rey

Ricardo Mejia

Rieke Kruse

Rob McGuire

Roland Fejes

Rosie Ettinger
and Colin Ettinger

Sam Carson
Sam Kimelman and
Jessica Kimelman

Sara Cox

Sarah Smith

Scott Newell

Sean and Elizabeth Murphy

Shan Wilkinson

Simon 'The Boff' Olliver

Stacy Fluegge

Stephanie Chapin

Steve Redmond,
Samantha Redmond
and Isabelle Redmond

Sullivan Robin Wells
and Griffin Raef Wells

Taryn Everdeen

Tiffany Jang Lydia Sochurek

Tim Handley

Tracey G. Tytko

Tracey James

Tyler Metzger

Vanessa

Valentine Ammeux

Vestin

Yann Dufour (For all
my family. Matthew
11:28-29, Psalms 23:2)

Yusaira

Zoe

This book is dedicated to my husband, Jon Wellstead, whose ability to sleep instantly and anywhere I envy and admire in equal measure. Thanks to the friends and family who supported me, even if they have never struggled with sleep themselves. A massive thank you to my collaborator Sophie: for being a joy to work with, and for using her talents to make this book a joy to look at. It is much, much better as a result of her involvement.

But most of all, thanks to the many strangers who took a risk, made a pledge and supported this book on Kickstarter. I hope that this finished book is even better than you hoped for, and that the tips inside help you to rediscover your ability to sleep easily and deeply for the rest of your life. I'd love to hear from you: sarah@mrandmscreative.com. In the meantime, good night and sleep tight. x

Sarah Plater